MY KETO
JOURNAL

Published by Mango Publishing Group, a division of Mango Media Inc.

Cover and Layout Design: Elina Diaz

For permission requests, please contact the publisher at:

Mango Publishing Group
2850 Douglas Road, 2nd Floor
Coral Gables, FL 33134 USA
info@mango.bz

For special orders, quantity sales, course adoptions and corporate sales, please email the publisher at sales@mango.bz. For trade and wholesale sales, please contact Ingram Publisher Services at customer.service@ingramcontent.com or +1.800.509.4887.

Medical resources: "Diet Review: Ketogenic Diet for Weight Loss." The Nutrition Source. May 07, 2018. Accessed November 2018. https://www.hsph.harvard.edu/nutritionsource/healthy-weight/diet-reviews/ketogenic-diet/

My Keto Journal: A Daily Food and Exercise Tracker to Help You Master Your Low-Carb, High-Fat, Ketogenic Diet

This book is not intended as an alternative or replacement to the medical advice of the reader's physicians. The reader should consult their doctor in all matters relating to their health prior to adjusting their diet.

Library of Congress Cataloging

ISBN: (print) 978-1-64250-027-1 (ebook) 978-1-64250-028-8
Library of Congress Control Number: Has ben applied for.
BISAC category code: SELF-HELP / Journaling HEALTH & FITNESS / Exercise
HEALTH & FITNESS / Diet & Nutrition / Weight Loss

Printed in the United States of America

MY KETO JOURNAL

A Daily Food and Exercise Tracker to Help You Master Your Low-Carb, High-Fat, Ketogenic Diet

Includes a 90-Day Meal and Activity Calendar

CORAL GABLES

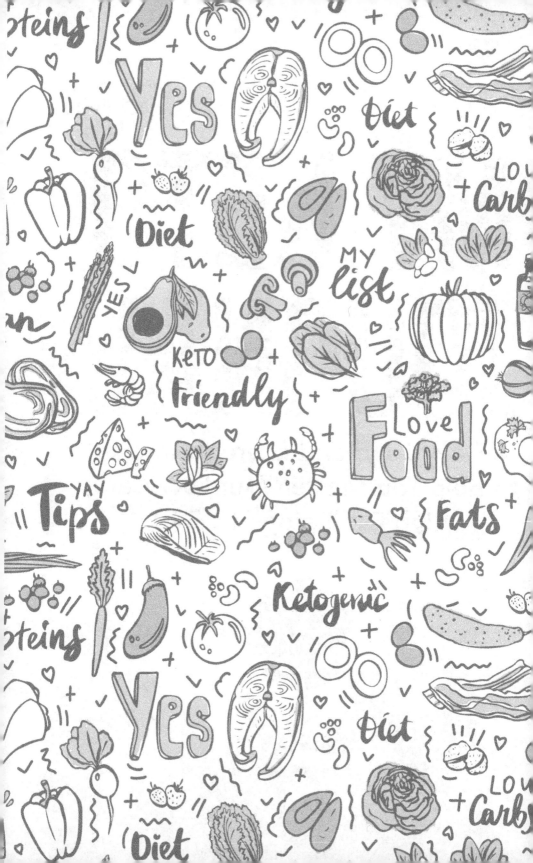

KETOGENESIS

[kee-toh-**jen**-uh-sis]

noun *Medicine/Medical*

1. the production of ketone bodies in the body, based on the idea of increasing fat consumption and adequate protein, while lowering carbohydrates and enabling the body to consume fats as fuel rather than carbohydrates.

BEFORE WE GET STARTED...

It is important to understand the science behind the method. When carbohydrates are consumed, our body transforms them into glucose. This is used to energize the body. But *how* you ask? As our glucose levels are increased, our pancreas will secrete insulin. Basically, this insulin is responsible for sending the glucose into our cells which then act as energy to help our body function.

Seems simple enough... Except that using carbohydrates as the main form of fuel for our bodies comes with health risks that vary from person to person.

But what if we did not feed our body glucose? When we limit the amount of carbohydrates that our body takes in, then our bodies will begin to convert *other* foods into fuel. This process is known as ketosis.

Think of ketosis as a switch that we can turn on and off in our bodies. It is managed by the foods we consume.

When used intelligently, this health practice can be incredibly beneficial in managing weight and energy levels. That is because, if we are not providing our bodies with carbohydrates, then our pancreas will create another hormone known as glucagon. Glucagon can then start to interact with our bodies by taking energy out of the stored fat we have by releasing it into our bloodstream.

THE KETO FLU

When you shock your body into a new eating regimen, you can expect it to respond in many different ways. While managing your weight and overall health is the main goal of introducing a ketogenic diet, there are other effects that might pop up.

During the first few days of shifting from a carbohydrate-fueled diet to keto-diet, it is normal for your body to feel confused, weak, and uncomfortable. Things like mental fog, fatigue, and anxiety are probable.

That does not mean that everyone will feel these, nor does it mean that you should not check with your doctor before starting a keto diet.

KETO BY THE NUMBERS

It will vary between person to person, but a good rule of thumb is:

Keto: 70% Fat, 25% Protein, 5% Carb

When transitioning in and out of keto, you can look to manage your macros accordingly. Again, it will vary from person to person, but a starting point can be near or at these numbers:

Starting or ending: 40% Fat, 55% Protein, 5% Carb

Some individuals see better results with a keto cycle while others prefer to stay on it exclusively. The secret is to find what works best for you as you work towards improving your health.

MY KETO KITCHEN

The big secret here is to lower your carbs and sugars and to eat foods that are higher in fat and protein. You want to stock your fridge and pantry with red meat, eggs, fish, chicken, vegetables, and natural fats like butter or olive oil. If in doubt, aim to eat foods that have less than 5% carbs.

Avoid sugar and starch at all costs. That means no to the 4 C's: cake, chocolate, cookies and candy. Other key items to avoid include fruit juices, sports drinks, sodas, and vitaminized waters. Read labels, as "healthy" foods like whole grain cereals and protein bars might be covered in unwanted sugars.

With an expanding market, keto-specific replacements are becoming more and more common. Keto breads, pastas, and rice now exist, allowing for an easier transition. But as always, remember to read the nutrition facts. You want there to be shorter ingredient lists and ideally very few, if any, processed foods.

MY KETO GOALS

List the goals you want to achieve every day as you embark on this new journey.

1. Eat keto, cleaner and healthier

2. Exercise

3. Love myself

4. _____

5. _____

6. _____

7. _____

8. _____

9. _____

10. _____

Fill in or circle the heart around each day that you achieve your goals.

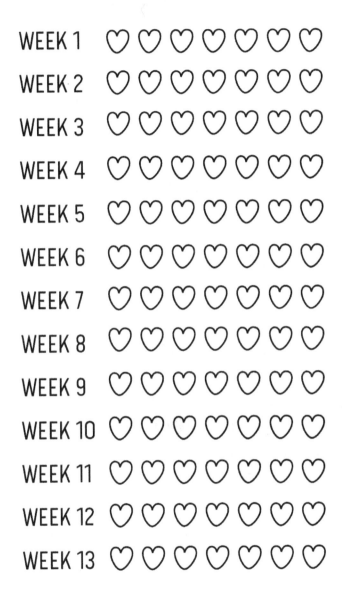

WEEK 1 ♡ ♡ ♡ ♡ ♡ ♡ ♡

WEEK 2 ♡ ♡ ♡ ♡ ♡ ♡ ♡

WEEK 3 ♡ ♡ ♡ ♡ ♡ ♡ ♡

WEEK 4 ♡ ♡ ♡ ♡ ♡ ♡ ♡

WEEK 5 ♡ ♡ ♡ ♡ ♡ ♡ ♡

WEEK 6 ♡ ♡ ♡ ♡ ♡ ♡ ♡

WEEK 7 ♡ ♡ ♡ ♡ ♡ ♡ ♡

WEEK 8 ♡ ♡ ♡ ♡ ♡ ♡ ♡

WEEK 9 ♡ ♡ ♡ ♡ ♡ ♡ ♡

WEEK 10 ♡ ♡ ♡ ♡ ♡ ♡ ♡

WEEK 11 ♡ ♡ ♡ ♡ ♡ ♡ ♡

WEEK 12 ♡ ♡ ♡ ♡ ♡ ♡ ♡

WEEK 13 ♡ ♡ ♡ ♡ ♡ ♡ ♡

LET'S GET MOVING!
MEASUREMENTS

CHEST: _____

BICEP: _____

WAIST: _____

HIP: _____

THIGHS: _____

CALVES: _____

WEIGHT: _____

HEART RATE: _____

BLOOD PRESSURE: _____

LET'S GET MOVING!
MEASUREMENTS

CHEST: _____

BICEP: _____

WAIST: _____

HIP: _____

THIGHS: _____

CALVES: _____

WEIGHT: _____

HEART RATE: _____

BLOOD PRESSURE: _____

HOW MANY HOURS OF SLEEP DID I GET? _____

BREAKFAST LUNCH DINNER

SNACKS

WATER

MACROS FOR THE DAY
CARBS: _____
PROTEIN: _____
FATS: _____
TOTAL CALORIES: _____

MY GOALS
1. EAT KETO, CLEANER AND HEALTHIER
2. EXERCISE
3. LOVE MYSELF
4.
5.
6.
7.
8.
9.
10.

ENERGY LEVEL

WORKOUT TRACKER

EXERCISE	REPS	SETS	WEIGHT	NOTES

HOW MANY HOURS OF SLEEP DID I GET? _____

BREAKFAST   LUNCH   DINNER

SNACKS

WATER

MACROS FOR THE DAY

CARBS: _____
PROTEIN: _____
FATS: _____
TOTAL CALORIES: _____

MY GOALS

1. EAT KETO, CLEANER AND HEALTHIER
2. EXERCISE
3. LOVE MYSELF
4.
5.
6.
7.
8.
9.
10.

ENERGY LEVEL

WORKOUT TRACKER

EXERCISE	REPS	SETS	WEIGHT	NOTES

DAY 3

BREAKFAST	LUNCH	DINNER

SNACKS

WATER

MACROS FOR THE DAY

CARBS: _____

PROTEIN: _____

FATS: _____

TOTAL CALORIES: _____

ENERGY LEVEL

MY GOALS

1. EAT KETO, CLEANER AND HEALTHIER
2. EXERCISE
3. LOVE MYSELF
4.
5.
6.
7.
8.
9.
10.

WORKOUT TRACKER

EXERCISE	REPS	SETS	WEIGHT	NOTES

HOW MANY HOURS OF SLEEP DID I GET? _____

BREAKFAST   LUNCH   DINNER

SNACKS

WATER

MACROS FOR THE DAY
CARBS: _____
PROTEIN: _____
FATS: _____
TOTAL CALORIES: _____

ENERGY LEVEL

MY GOALS
1. EAT KETO, CLEANER AND HEALTHIER
2. EXERCISE
3. LOVE MYSELF
4.
5.
6.
7.
8.
9.
10.

WORKOUT TRACKER

EXERCISE	REPS	SETS	WEIGHT	NOTES

BREAKFAST   LUNCH   DINNER

SNACKS

WATER

MACROS FOR THE DAY

CARBS: _____

PROTEIN: _____

FATS: _____

TOTAL CALORIES: _____

ENERGY LEVEL

MY GOALS

1. EAT KETO, CLEANER AND HEALTHIER

2. EXERCISE

3. LOVE MYSELF

4.

5.

6.

7.

8.

9.

10.

WORKOUT TRACKER

EXERCISE	REPS	SETS	WEIGHT	NOTES

HOW MANY HOURS OF SLEEP DID I GET? _____

BREAKFAST   LUNCH   DINNER

SNACKS

WATER

MACROS FOR THE DAY
CARBS: _____
PROTEIN: _____
FATS: _____
TOTAL CALORIES: _____

MY GOALS
1. EAT KETO, CLEANER AND HEALTHIER
2. EXERCISE
3. LOVE MYSELF
4.
5.
6.
7.
8.
9.
10.

ENERGY LEVEL

WORKOUT TRACKER

EXERCISE	REPS	SETS	WEIGHT	NOTES

HOW MANY HOURS OF SLEEP DID I GET? _____

BREAKFAST	LUNCH	DINNER

SNACKS

WATER

MACROS FOR THE DAY
CARBS: _____
PROTEIN: _____
FATS: _____
TOTAL CALORIES: _____

MY GOALS
1. EAT KETO, CLEANER AND HEALTHIER
2. EXERCISE
3. LOVE MYSELF
4.
5.
6.
7.
8.
9.
10.

ENERGY LEVEL

WORKOUT TRACKER

EXERCISE	REPS	SETS	WEIGHT	NOTES

HOW MANY HOURS OF SLEEP DID I GET? _____

| BREAKFAST | LUNCH | DINNER |

SNACKS

WATER

MACROS FOR THE DAY

CARBS: _____
PROTEIN: _____
FATS: _____
TOTAL CALORIES: _____

ENERGY LEVEL

MY GOALS

1. EAT KETO, CLEANER AND HEALTHIER
2. EXERCISE
3. LOVE MYSELF
4.
5.
6.
7.
8.
9.
10.

WORKOUT TRACKER

EXERCISE	REPS	SETS	WEIGHT	NOTES

DAY 9

BREAKFAST	LUNCH	DINNER

SNACKS

WATER

MACROS FOR THE DAY

CARBS: _____
PROTEIN: _____
FATS: _____
TOTAL CALORIES: _____

ENERGY LEVEL

MY GOALS

1. EAT KETO, CLEANER AND HEALTHIER
2. EXERCISE
3. LOVE MYSELF
4.
5.
6.
7.
8.
9.
10.

WORKOUT TRACKER

EXERCISE	REPS	SETS	WEIGHT	NOTES

HOW MANY HOURS OF SLEEP DID I GET? _____

BREAKFAST

LUNCH

DINNER

SNACKS

WATER

MACROS FOR THE DAY

CARBS: _____
PROTEIN: _____
FATS: _____
TOTAL CALORIES: _____

MY GOALS

1. EAT KETO, CLEANER AND HEALTHIER
2. EXERCISE
3. LOVE MYSELF
4.
5.
6.
7.
8.
9.
10.

ENERGY LEVEL

WORKOUT TRACKER

EXERCISE	REPS	SETS	WEIGHT	NOTES

DAY 11   **HOW MANY HOURS OF SLEEP DID I GET?** _____

BREAKFAST	LUNCH	DINNER

SNACKS

WATER

MACROS FOR THE DAY
CARBS: _____
PROTEIN: _____
FATS: _____
TOTAL CALORIES: _____

MY GOALS
1. EAT KETO, CLEANER AND HEALTHIER
2. EXERCISE
3. LOVE MYSELF
4.
5.
6.
7.
8.
9.
10.

ENERGY LEVEL

WORKOUT TRACKER

EXERCISE	REPS	SETS	WEIGHT	NOTES

BREAKFAST	LUNCH	DINNER

SNACKS

WATER

MACROS FOR THE DAY

CARBS: _____
PROTEIN: _____
FATS: _____
TOTAL CALORIES: _____

MY GOALS

1. EAT KETO, CLEANER AND HEALTHIER
2. EXERCISE
3. LOVE MYSELF
4.
5.
6.
7.
8.
9.
10.

ENERGY LEVEL

WORKOUT TRACKER

EXERCISE	REPS	SETS	WEIGHT	NOTES

BREAKFAST	**LUNCH**	**DINNER**

SNACKS

WATER

MACROS FOR THE DAY

CARBS: _____

PROTEIN: _____

FATS: _____

TOTAL CALORIES: _____

ENERGY LEVEL

MY GOALS

1. EAT KETO, CLEANER AND HEALTHIER

2. EXERCISE

3. LOVE MYSELF

4.

5.

6.

7.

8.

9.

10.

WORKOUT TRACKER

EXERCISE	REPS	SETS	WEIGHT	NOTES

HOW MANY HOURS OF SLEEP DID I GET? _____

BREAKFAST   **LUNCH**   **DINNER**

SNACKS

WATER

MACROS FOR THE DAY

CARBS: _____
PROTEIN: _____
FATS: _____
TOTAL CALORIES: _____

ENERGY LEVEL

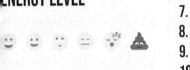

MY GOALS

1. EAT KETO, CLEANER AND HEALTHIER
2. EXERCISE
3. LOVE MYSELF
4.
5.
6.
7.
8.
9.
10.

WORKOUT TRACKER

EXERCISE	REPS	SETS	WEIGHT	NOTES

HOW MANY HOURS OF SLEEP DID I GET? _____

BREAKFAST	LUNCH	DINNER

SNACKS

WATER

MACROS FOR THE DAY

CARBS: _____

PROTEIN: _____

FATS: _____

TOTAL CALORIES: _____

MY GOALS

1. EAT KETO, CLEANER AND HEALTHIER

2. EXERCISE

3. LOVE MYSELF

4.

5.

6.

7.

8.

9.

10.

ENERGY LEVEL

😀 😄 😐 😑 😴 💩

WORKOUT TRACKER

EXERCISE	REPS	SETS	WEIGHT	NOTES

BREAKFAST	LUNCH	DINNER

SNACKS

WATER

MACROS FOR THE DAY

CARBS: _____

PROTEIN: _____

FATS: _____

TOTAL CALORIES: _____

MY GOALS

1. EAT KETO, CLEANER AND HEALTHIER
2. EXERCISE
3. LOVE MYSELF
4.
5.
6.
7.
8.
9.
10.

ENERGY LEVEL

WORKOUT TRACKER

EXERCISE	REPS	SETS	WEIGHT	NOTES

HOW MANY HOURS OF SLEEP DID I GET? _____

BREAKFAST	LUNCH	DINNER

SNACKS

WATER

MACROS FOR THE DAY
CARBS: _____
PROTEIN: _____
FATS: _____
TOTAL CALORIES: _____

ENERGY LEVEL

MY GOALS
1. EAT KETO, CLEANER AND HEALTHIER
2. EXERCISE
3. LOVE MYSELF
4.
5.
6.
7.
8.
9.
10.

WORKOUT TRACKER

EXERCISE	REPS	SETS	WEIGHT	NOTES

HOW MANY HOURS OF SLEEP DID I GET? _____

BREAKFAST	LUNCH	DINNER

SNACKS

WATER

MACROS FOR THE DAY

CARBS: _____
PROTEIN: _____
FATS: _____
TOTAL CALORIES: _____

MY GOALS

1. EAT KETO, CLEANER AND HEALTHIER
2. EXERCISE
3. LOVE MYSELF
4.
5.
6.
7.
8.
9.
10.

ENERGY LEVEL

WORKOUT TRACKER

EXERCISE	REPS	SETS	WEIGHT	NOTES

DAY 19   **HOW MANY HOURS OF SLEEP DID I GET?** _____

BREAKFAST	**LUNCH**	**DINNER**

SNACKS

WATER

MACROS FOR THE DAY
CARBS: _____
PROTEIN: _____
FATS: _____
TOTAL CALORIES: _____

MY GOALS
1. EAT KETO, CLEANER AND HEALTHIER
2. EXERCISE
3. LOVE MYSELF
4.
5.
6.
7.
8.
9.
10.

ENERGY LEVEL

WORKOUT TRACKER

EXERCISE	REPS	SETS	WEIGHT	NOTES

HOW MANY HOURS OF SLEEP DID I GET? _____

BREAKFAST   **LUNCH**   **DINNER**

SNACKS

WATER

MACROS FOR THE DAY   **MY GOALS**
  CARBS: _____   **1.** EAT KETO, CLEANER AND HEALTHIER
  PROTEIN: _____   **2.** EXERCISE
  FATS: _____   **3.** LOVE MYSELF
  TOTAL CALORIES: _____   **4.**
                              5.
ENERGY LEVEL   **6.**
                              7.
😄 😊 😕 😐 😴 💩   **8.**
                              9.
                              10.

WORKOUT TRACKER

EXERCISE	REPS	SETS	WEIGHT	NOTES

HOW MANY HOURS OF SLEEP DID I GET? _____

BREAKFAST	LUNCH	DINNER

SNACKS

WATER

MACROS FOR THE DAY

CARBS: _____
PROTEIN: _____
FATS: _____
TOTAL CALORIES: _____

MY GOALS

1. EAT KETO, CLEANER AND HEALTHIER
2. EXERCISE
3. LOVE MYSELF
4.
5.
6.
7.
8.
9.
10.

ENERGY LEVEL

WORKOUT TRACKER

EXERCISE	REPS	SETS	WEIGHT	NOTES

HOW MANY HOURS OF SLEEP DID I GET? _____

BREAKFAST	LUNCH	DINNER

SNACKS

WATER

MACROS FOR THE DAY
CARBS: _____
PROTEIN: _____
FATS: _____
TOTAL CALORIES: _____

MY GOALS
1. EAT KETO, CLEANER AND HEALTHIER
2. EXERCISE
3. LOVE MYSELF
4.
5.
6.
7.
8.
9.
10.

ENERGY LEVEL

WORKOUT TRACKER

EXERCISE	REPS	SETS	WEIGHT	NOTES

HOW MANY HOURS OF SLEEP DID I GET? _____

BREAKFAST	LUNCH	DINNER

SNACKS

WATER

MACROS FOR THE DAY

CARBS: _____
PROTEIN: _____
FATS: _____
TOTAL CALORIES: _____

MY GOALS

1. EAT KETO, CLEANER AND HEALTHIER
2. EXERCISE
3. LOVE MYSELF
4.
5.
6.
7.
8.
9.
10.

ENERGY LEVEL

WORKOUT TRACKER

EXERCISE	REPS	SETS	WEIGHT	NOTES

HOW MANY HOURS OF SLEEP DID I GET? _____

BREAKFAST	LUNCH	DINNER

SNACKS

WATER

MACROS FOR THE DAY

CARBS: _____
PROTEIN: _____
FATS: _____
TOTAL CALORIES: _____

MY GOALS

1. EAT KETO, CLEANER AND HEALTHIER
2. EXERCISE
3. LOVE MYSELF
4.
5.
6.
7.
8.
9.
10.

ENERGY LEVEL

WORKOUT TRACKER

EXERCISE	REPS	SETS	WEIGHT	NOTES

BREAKFAST	LUNCH	DINNER

SNACKS

WATER

MACROS FOR THE DAY

CARBS: _____
PROTEIN: _____
FATS: _____
TOTAL CALORIES: _____

ENERGY LEVEL

MY GOALS

1. EAT KETO, CLEANER AND HEALTHIER
2. EXERCISE
3. LOVE MYSELF
4.
5.
6.
7.
8.
9.
10.

WORKOUT TRACKER

EXERCISE	REPS	SETS	WEIGHT	NOTES

HOW MANY HOURS OF SLEEP DID I GET? _____

BREAKFAST   LUNCH   DINNER

SNACKS

WATER

MACROS FOR THE DAY

CARBS: _____
PROTEIN: _____
FATS: _____
TOTAL CALORIES: _____

MY GOALS

1. EAT KETO, CLEANER AND HEALTHIER
2. EXERCISE
3. LOVE MYSELF
4.
5.
6.
7.
8.
9.
10.

ENERGY LEVEL

😄 😊 🙁 😐 😴 💩

WORKOUT TRACKER

EXERCISE	REPS	SETS	WEIGHT	NOTES

HOW MANY HOURS OF SLEEP DID I GET? _____

BREAKFAST	LUNCH	DINNER

SNACKS

WATER

MACROS FOR THE DAY

CARBS: _____

PROTEIN: _____

FATS: _____

TOTAL CALORIES: _____

MY GOALS

1. EAT KETO, CLEANER AND HEALTHIER
2. EXERCISE
3. LOVE MYSELF
4.
5.
6.
7.
8.
9.
10.

ENERGY LEVEL

WORKOUT TRACKER

EXERCISE	REPS	SETS	WEIGHT	NOTES

HOW MANY HOURS OF SLEEP DID I GET? _____

BREAKFAST	LUNCH	DINNER

SNACKS

WATER

MACROS FOR THE DAY

CARBS: _____
PROTEIN: _____
FATS: _____
TOTAL CALORIES: _____

MY GOALS

1. EAT KETO, CLEANER AND HEALTHIER
2. EXERCISE
3. LOVE MYSELF
4.
5.
6.
7.
8.
9.
10.

ENERGY LEVEL

WORKOUT TRACKER

EXERCISE	REPS	SETS	WEIGHT	NOTES

BREAKFAST   LUNCH   DINNER

SNACKS

WATER

MACROS FOR THE DAY

CARBS: _____
PROTEIN: _____
FATS: _____
TOTAL CALORIES: _____

ENERGY LEVEL

😃 😊 😕 😑 😴 💩

MY GOALS

1. EAT KETO, CLEANER AND HEALTHIER
2. EXERCISE
3. LOVE MYSELF
4.
5.
6.
7.
8.
9.
10.

WORKOUT TRACKER

EXERCISE	REPS	SETS	WEIGHT	NOTES

HOW MANY HOURS OF SLEEP DID I GET? _____

BREAKFAST	LUNCH	DINNER

SNACKS

WATER

MACROS FOR THE DAY

CARBS: _____
PROTEIN: _____
FATS: _____
TOTAL CALORIES: _____

MY GOALS

1. EAT KETO, CLEANER AND HEALTHIER
2. EXERCISE
3. LOVE MYSELF
4.
5.
6.
7.
8.
9.
10.

ENERGY LEVEL

WORKOUT TRACKER

EXERCISE	REPS	SETS	WEIGHT	NOTES

HOW MANY HOURS OF SLEEP DID I GET? _____

BREAKFAST	LUNCH	DINNER

SNACKS

WATER

MACROS FOR THE DAY

CARBS: _____

PROTEIN: _____

FATS: _____

TOTAL CALORIES: _____

ENERGY LEVEL

MY GOALS

1. EAT KETO, CLEANER AND HEALTHIER

2. EXERCISE

3. LOVE MYSELF

4.

5.

6.

7.

8.

9.

10.

WORKOUT TRACKER

EXERCISE	REPS	SETS	WEIGHT	NOTES

HOW MANY HOURS OF SLEEP DID I GET? _____

BREAKFAST	LUNCH	DINNER

SNACKS

WATER

MACROS FOR THE DAY

CARBS: _____
PROTEIN: _____
FATS: _____
TOTAL CALORIES: _____

ENERGY LEVEL

MY GOALS

1. EAT KETO, CLEANER AND HEALTHIER
2. EXERCISE
3. LOVE MYSELF
4.
5.
6.
7.
8.
9.
10.

WORKOUT TRACKER

EXERCISE	REPS	SETS	WEIGHT	NOTES

HOW MANY HOURS OF SLEEP DID I GET? _____

BREAKFAST	LUNCH	DINNER

SNACKS

WATER

MACROS FOR THE DAY

CARBS: _____

PROTEIN: _____

FATS: _____

TOTAL CALORIES: _____

MY GOALS

1. EAT KETO, CLEANER AND HEALTHIER

2. EXERCISE

3. LOVE MYSELF

4.

5.

6.

7.

8.

9.

10.

ENERGY LEVEL

😄 😊 🙁 😐 😴 💩

WORKOUT TRACKER

EXERCISE	REPS	SETS	WEIGHT	NOTES

HOW MANY HOURS OF SLEEP DID I GET? _____

BREAKFAST	LUNCH	DINNER

SNACKS

WATER

MACROS FOR THE DAY

CARBS: _____

PROTEIN: _____

FATS: _____

TOTAL CALORIES: _____

MY GOALS

1. EAT KETO, CLEANER AND HEALTHIER

2. EXERCISE

3. LOVE MYSELF

4.

5.

6.

7.

8.

9.

10.

ENERGY LEVEL

WORKOUT TRACKER

EXERCISE	REPS	SETS	WEIGHT	NOTES

HOW MANY HOURS OF SLEEP DID I GET? _____

BREAKFAST	**LUNCH**	**DINNER**

SNACKS

WATER

MACROS FOR THE DAY
CARBS: _____
PROTEIN: _____
FATS: _____
TOTAL CALORIES: _____

MY GOALS
1. EAT KETO, CLEANER AND HEALTHIER
2. EXERCISE
3. LOVE MYSELF
4.
5.
6.
7.
8.
9.
10.

ENERGY LEVEL

WORKOUT TRACKER

EXERCISE	REPS	SETS	WEIGHT	NOTES

BREAKFAST	**LUNCH**	**DINNER**

SNACKS

WATER

MACROS FOR THE DAY

CARBS: _____

PROTEIN: _____

FATS: _____

TOTAL CALORIES: _____

MY GOALS

1. EAT KETO, CLEANER AND HEALTHIER
2. EXERCISE
3. LOVE MYSELF
4.
5.
6.
7.
8.
9.
10.

ENERGY LEVEL

😊 😄 😐 😑 😴 💩

WORKOUT TRACKER

EXERCISE	REPS	SETS	WEIGHT	NOTES

HOW MANY HOURS OF SLEEP DID I GET? _____

BREAKFAST	**LUNCH**	**DINNER**

SNACKS

WATER

MACROS FOR THE DAY
CARBS: _____
PROTEIN: _____
FATS: _____
TOTAL CALORIES: _____

MY GOALS
1. EAT KETO, CLEANER AND HEALTHIER
2. EXERCISE
3. LOVE MYSELF
4.
5.
6.
7.
8.
9.
10.

ENERGY LEVEL

WORKOUT TRACKER

EXERCISE	REPS	SETS	WEIGHT	NOTES

BREAKFAST	LUNCH	DINNER

SNACKS

WATER

MACROS FOR THE DAY

CARBS: _____
PROTEIN: _____
FATS: _____
TOTAL CALORIES: _____

ENERGY LEVEL

 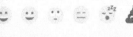

MY GOALS

1. EAT KETO, CLEANER AND HEALTHIER
2. EXERCISE
3. LOVE MYSELF
4.
5.
6.
7.
8.
9.
10.

WORKOUT TRACKER

EXERCISE	REPS	SETS	WEIGHT	NOTES

HOW MANY HOURS OF SLEEP DID I GET? _____

BREAKFAST	**LUNCH**	**DINNER**

SNACKS

WATER

MACROS FOR THE DAY

CARBS: _____
PROTEIN: _____
FATS: _____
TOTAL CALORIES: _____

MY GOALS

1. EAT KETO, CLEANER AND HEALTHIER
2. EXERCISE
3. LOVE MYSELF
4.
5.
6.
7.
8.
9.
10.

ENERGY LEVEL

WORKOUT TRACKER

EXERCISE	REPS	SETS	WEIGHT	NOTES

HOW MANY HOURS OF SLEEP DID I GET? _____

BREAKFAST	**LUNCH**	**DINNER**

SNACKS

WATER

MACROS FOR THE DAY

CARBS: _____

PROTEIN: _____

FATS: _____

TOTAL CALORIES: _____

MY GOALS

1. EAT KETO, CLEANER AND HEALTHIER
2. EXERCISE
3. LOVE MYSELF
4.
5.
6.
7.
8.
9.
10.

ENERGY LEVEL

😊 😃 🙂 😐 😴 💩

WORKOUT TRACKER

EXERCISE	REPS	SETS	WEIGHT	NOTES

DAY 41   **HOW MANY HOURS OF SLEEP DID I GET?** _____

BREAKFAST	**LUNCH**	**DINNER**

SNACKS

WATER

MACROS FOR THE DAY

CARBS: _____
PROTEIN: _____
FATS: _____
TOTAL CALORIES: _____

ENERGY LEVEL

😄 😊 🙁 😩 😴 💩

MY GOALS

1. EAT KETO, CLEANER AND HEALTHIER
2. EXERCISE
3. LOVE MYSELF
4.
5.
6.
7.
8.
9.
10.

WORKOUT TRACKER

EXERCISE	REPS	SETS	WEIGHT	NOTES

HOW MANY HOURS OF SLEEP DID I GET? _____

BREAKFAST	LUNCH	DINNER

NACKS

VATER

MACROS FOR THE DAY

CARBS: _____

PROTEIN: _____

FATS: _____

TOTAL CALORIES: _____

ENERGY LEVEL

 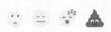

MY GOALS

1. EAT KETO, CLEANER AND HEALTHIER

2. EXERCISE

3. LOVE MYSELF

4.

5.

6.

7.

8.

9.

10.

WORKOUT TRACKER

EXERCISE	REPS	SETS	WEIGHT	NOTES

DAY 43   HOW MANY HOURS OF SLEEP DID I GET? _____

BREAKFAST	LUNCH	DINNER

SNACKS

WATER

MACROS FOR THE DAY
CARBS: _____
PROTEIN: _____
FATS: _____
TOTAL CALORIES: _____

ENERGY LEVEL

MY GOALS
1. EAT KETO, CLEANER AND HEALTHIER
2. EXERCISE
3. LOVE MYSELF
4.
5.
6.
7.
8.
9.
10.

WORKOUT TRACKER

EXERCISE	REPS	SETS	WEIGHT	NOTES

HOW MANY HOURS OF SLEEP DID I GET? _____

BREAKFAST   LUNCH   DINNER

SNACKS

WATER

MACROS FOR THE DAY
CARBS: _____
PROTEIN: _____
FATS: _____
TOTAL CALORIES: _____

MY GOALS
1. EAT KETO, CLEANER AND HEALTHIER
2. EXERCISE
3. LOVE MYSELF
4.
5.
6.
7.
8.
9.
10.

ENERGY LEVEL

 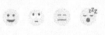

WORKOUT TRACKER

EXERCISE	REPS	SETS	WEIGHT	NOTES

DAY 45

BREAKFAST	LUNCH	DINNER

SNACKS

WATER

MACROS FOR THE DAY

CARBS: _____

PROTEIN: _____

FATS: _____

TOTAL CALORIES: _____

ENERGY LEVEL

MY GOALS

1. EAT KETO, CLEANER AND HEALTHIER

2. EXERCISE

3. LOVE MYSELF

4.

5.

6.

7.

8.

9.

10.

WORKOUT TRACKER

EXERCISE	REPS	SETS	WEIGHT	NOTES

LET'S KEEP GOING!
MEASUREMENTS

CHEST: _____

BICEP: _____

WAIST: _____

HIP: _____

THIGHS: _____

CALVES: _____

WEIGHT: _____

HEART RATE: _____

BLOOD PRESSURE: _____

LET'S KEEP GOING!
MEASUREMENTS

CHEST: _____

BICEP: _____

WAIST: _____

HIP: _____

THIGHS: _____

CALVES: _____

WEIGHT: _____

HEART RATE: _____

BLOOD PRESSURE: _____

HOW MANY HOURS OF SLEEP DID I GET? _____

BREAKFAST   LUNCH   DINNER

SNACKS

WATER

MACROS FOR THE DAY

CARBS: _____
PROTEIN: _____
FATS: _____
TOTAL CALORIES: _____

MY GOALS

1. EAT KETO, CLEANER AND HEALTHIER
2. EXERCISE
3. LOVE MYSELF
4.
5.
6.
7.
8.
9.
10.

ENERGY LEVEL

WORKOUT TRACKER

EXERCISE	REPS	SETS	WEIGHT	NOTES

HOW MANY HOURS OF SLEEP DID I GET? _____

BREAKFAST	LUNCH	DINNER

SNACKS

WATER

MACROS FOR THE DAY

CARBS: _____
PROTEIN: _____
FATS: _____
TOTAL CALORIES: _____

MY GOALS

1. EAT KETO, CLEANER AND HEALTHIER
2. EXERCISE
3. LOVE MYSELF
4.
5.
6.
7.
8.
9.
10.

ENERGY LEVEL

WORKOUT TRACKER

EXERCISE	REPS	SETS	WEIGHT	NOTES

HOW MANY HOURS OF SLEEP DID I GET? _____

BREAKFAST	LUNCH	DINNER

SNACKS

WATER

MACROS FOR THE DAY
CARBS: _____
PROTEIN: _____
FATS: _____
TOTAL CALORIES: _____

MY GOALS
1. EAT KETO, CLEANER AND HEALTHIER
2. EXERCISE
3. LOVE MYSELF
4.
5.
6.
7.
8.
9.
10.

ENERGY LEVEL

WORKOUT TRACKER

EXERCISE	REPS	SETS	WEIGHT	NOTES

HOW MANY HOURS OF SLEEP DID I GET? _____

BREAKFAST   LUNCH   DINNER

SNACKS

WATER

MACROS FOR THE DAY

CARBS: _____
PROTEIN: _____
FATS: _____
TOTAL CALORIES: _____

MY GOALS

1. EAT KETO, CLEANER AND HEALTHIER
2. EXERCISE
3. LOVE MYSELF
4.
5.
6.
7.
8.
9.
10.

ENERGY LEVEL

WORKOUT TRACKER

EXERCISE	REPS	SETS	WEIGHT	NOTES

HOW MANY HOURS OF SLEEP DID I GET? _____

BREAKFAST	**LUNCH**	**DINNER**

SNACKS

WATER

MACROS FOR THE DAY

CARBS: _____
PROTEIN: _____
FATS: _____
TOTAL CALORIES: _____

MY GOALS

1. EAT KETO, CLEANER AND HEALTHIER
2. EXERCISE
3. LOVE MYSELF
4.
5.
6.
7.
8.
9.
10.

ENERGY LEVEL

😃 😄 😕 😐 😴 💩

WORKOUT TRACKER

EXERCISE	REPS	SETS	WEIGHT	NOTES

HOW MANY HOURS OF SLEEP DID I GET? _____

BREAKFAST	LUNCH	DINNER

SNACKS

WATER

MACROS FOR THE DAY
CARBS: _____
PROTEIN: _____
FATS: _____
TOTAL CALORIES: _____

MY GOALS
1. EAT KETO, CLEANER AND HEALTHIER
2. EXERCISE
3. LOVE MYSELF
4.
5.
6.
7.
8.
9.
10.

ENERGY LEVEL

WORKOUT TRACKER

EXERCISE	REPS	SETS	WEIGHT	NOTES

BREAKFAST	LUNCH	DINNER

NACKS

VATER

MACROS FOR THE DAY

CARBS: _____

PROTEIN: _____

FATS: _____

TOTAL CALORIES: _____

ENERGY LEVEL

😊 😄 😕 😐 😴 💩

MY GOALS

1. EAT KETO, CLEANER AND HEALTHIER

2. EXERCISE

3. LOVE MYSELF

4.

5.

6.

7.

8.

9.

10.

WORKOUT TRACKER

EXERCISE	REPS	SETS	WEIGHT	NOTES

HOW MANY HOURS OF SLEEP DID I GET? _____

BREAKFAST	LUNCH	DINNER

SNACKS

WATER

MACROS FOR THE DAY

CARBS: _____
PROTEIN: _____
FATS: _____
TOTAL CALORIES: _____

ENERGY LEVEL

MY GOALS

1. EAT KETO, CLEANER AND HEALTHIER
2. EXERCISE
3. LOVE MYSELF
4.
5.
6.
7.
8.
9.
10.

WORKOUT TRACKER

EXERCISE	REPS	SETS	WEIGHT	NOTES

HOW MANY HOURS OF SLEEP DID I GET? _____

| BREAKFAST | LUNCH | DINNER |

SNACKS

WATER

MACROS FOR THE DAY

CARBS: _____
PROTEIN: _____
FATS: _____
TOTAL CALORIES: _____

ENERGY LEVEL

😊 😄 🙁 😑 😴 💩

MY GOALS

1. EAT KETO, CLEANER AND HEALTHIER
2. EXERCISE
3. LOVE MYSELF
4.
5.
6.
7.
8.
9.
10.

WORKOUT TRACKER

EXERCISE	REPS	SETS	WEIGHT	NOTES

DAY 56   HOW MANY HOURS OF SLEEP DID I GET? _____

| BREAKFAST | LUNCH | DINNER |

SNACKS

WATER

MACROS FOR THE DAY
CARBS: _____
PROTEIN: _____
FATS: _____
TOTAL CALORIES: _____

MY GOALS
1. EAT KETO, CLEANER AND HEALTHIER
2. EXERCISE
3. LOVE MYSELF
4.
5.
6.
7.
8.
9.
10.

ENERGY LEVEL

WORKOUT TRACKER

EXERCISE	REPS	SETS	WEIGHT	NOTES

HOW MANY HOURS OF SLEEP DID I GET? _____

BREAKFAST	LUNCH	DINNER

SNACKS

WATER

MACROS FOR THE DAY

CARBS: _____

PROTEIN: _____

FATS: _____

TOTAL CALORIES: _____

MY GOALS

1. EAT KETO, CLEANER AND HEALTHIER
2. EXERCISE
3. LOVE MYSELF
4.
5.
6.
7.
8.
9.
10.

ENERGY LEVEL

WORKOUT TRACKER

EXERCISE	REPS	SETS	WEIGHT	NOTES

BREAKFAST	LUNCH	DINNER

SNACKS

WATER

MACROS FOR THE DAY
CARBS: _____
PROTEIN: _____
FATS: _____
TOTAL CALORIES: _____

ENERGY LEVEL

MY GOALS
1. EAT KETO, CLEANER AND HEALTHIER
2. EXERCISE
3. LOVE MYSELF
4.
5.
6.
7.
8.
9.
10.

WORKOUT TRACKER

EXERCISE	REPS	SETS	WEIGHT	NOTES

BREAKFAST	LUNCH	DINNER

SNACKS

WATER

MACROS FOR THE DAY

CARBS: _____
PROTEIN: _____
FATS: _____
TOTAL CALORIES: _____

ENERGY LEVEL

 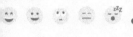

MY GOALS

1. EAT KETO, CLEANER AND HEALTHIER
2. EXERCISE
3. LOVE MYSELF
4.
5.
6.
7.
8.
9.
10.

WORKOUT TRACKER

EXERCISE	REPS	SETS	WEIGHT	NOTES

DAY 60

HOW MANY HOURS OF SLEEP DID I GET? _____

BREAKFAST

LUNCH

DINNER

SNACKS

WATER

MACROS FOR THE DAY

CARBS: _____

PROTEIN: _____

FATS: _____

TOTAL CALORIES: _____

MY GOALS

1. EAT KETO, CLEANER AND HEALTHIER
2. EXERCISE
3. LOVE MYSELF
4.
5.
6.
7.
8.
9.
10.

ENERGY LEVEL

WORKOUT TRACKER

EXERCISE	REPS	SETS	WEIGHT	NOTES

HOW MANY HOURS OF SLEEP DID I GET? _____

BREAKFAST	**LUNCH**	**DINNER**

NACKS

VATER

MACROS FOR THE DAY

CARBS: _____

PROTEIN: _____

FATS: _____

TOTAL CALORIES: _____

ENERGY LEVEL

MY GOALS

1. EAT KETO, CLEANER AND HEALTHIER

2. EXERCISE

3. LOVE MYSELF

4.

5.

6.

7.

8.

9.

10.

WORKOUT TRACKER

EXERCISE	REPS	SETS	WEIGHT	NOTES

DAY 62

BREAKFAST	LUNCH	DINNER

SNACKS

WATER

MACROS FOR THE DAY

CARBS: _____

PROTEIN: _____

FATS: _____

TOTAL CALORIES: _____

ENERGY LEVEL

MY GOALS

1. EAT KETO, CLEANER AND HEALTHIER

2. EXERCISE

3. LOVE MYSELF

4.

5.

6.

7.

8.

9.

10.

WORKOUT TRACKER

EXERCISE	REPS	SETS	WEIGHT	NOTES

HOW MANY HOURS OF SLEEP DID I GET? _____

BREAKFAST	LUNCH	DINNER

SNACKS

WATER

MACROS FOR THE DAY

CARBS: _____
PROTEIN: _____
FATS: _____
TOTAL CALORIES: _____

MY GOALS

1. EAT KETO, CLEANER AND HEALTHIER
2. EXERCISE
3. LOVE MYSELF
4.
5.
6.
7.
8.
9.
10.

ENERGY LEVEL

WORKOUT TRACKER

EXERCISE	REPS	SETS	WEIGHT	NOTES

HOW MANY HOURS OF SLEEP DID I GET? _____

BREAKFAST   LUNCH   DINNER

SNACKS

WATER

MACROS FOR THE DAY

CARBS: _____
PROTEIN: _____
FATS: _____
TOTAL CALORIES: _____

ENERGY LEVEL

MY GOALS

1. EAT KETO, CLEANER AND HEALTHIER
2. EXERCISE
3. LOVE MYSELF
4.
5.
6.
7.
8.
9.
10.

WORKOUT TRACKER

EXERCISE	REPS	SETS	WEIGHT	NOTES

BREAKFAST   LUNCH   DINNER

NACKS

ATER

ACROS FOR THE DAY   MY GOALS

CARBS: _____
PROTEIN: _____
FATS: _____
TOTAL CALORIES: _____

NERGY LEVEL

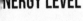 

MY GOALS
1. EAT KETO, CLEANER AND HEALTHIER
2. EXERCISE
3. LOVE MYSELF
4.
5.
6.
7.
8.
9.
10.

ORKOUT TRACKER

EXERCISE	REPS	SETS	WEIGHT	NOTES

BREAKFAST	LUNCH	DINNER

SNACKS

WATER

MACROS FOR THE DAY

CARBS: _____

PROTEIN: _____

FATS: _____

TOTAL CALORIES: _____

ENERGY LEVEL

MY GOALS

1. EAT KETO, CLEANER AND HEALTHIER

2. EXERCISE

3. LOVE MYSELF

4.

5.

6.

7.

8.

9.

10.

WORKOUT TRACKER

EXERCISE	REPS	SETS	WEIGHT	NOTES

HOW MANY HOURS OF SLEEP DID I GET? _____

BREAKFAST	LUNCH	DINNER

SNACKS

WATER

MACROS FOR THE DAY

CARBS: _____
PROTEIN: _____
FATS: _____
TOTAL CALORIES: _____

ENERGY LEVEL

😃 😄 🙂 😐 😴 💩

MY GOALS

1. EAT KETO, CLEANER AND HEALTHIER
2. EXERCISE
3. LOVE MYSELF
4.
5.
6.
7.
8.
9.
10.

WORKOUT TRACKER

EXERCISE	REPS	SETS	WEIGHT	NOTES

HOW MANY HOURS OF SLEEP DID I GET? _____

BREAKFAST	LUNCH	DINNER

SNACKS

WATER

MACROS FOR THE DAY

CARBS: _____
PROTEIN: _____
FATS: _____
TOTAL CALORIES: _____

MY GOALS

1. EAT KETO, CLEANER AND HEALTHIER
2. EXERCISE
3. LOVE MYSELF
4.
5.
6.
7.
8.
9.
10.

ENERGY LEVEL

WORKOUT TRACKER

EXERCISE	REPS	SETS	WEIGHT	NOTES

| BREAKFAST | LUNCH | DINNER |

NACKS

VATER

MACROS FOR THE DAY
CARBS: _____
PROTEIN: _____
FATS: _____
TOTAL CALORIES: _____

ENERGY LEVEL

 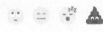

MY GOALS
1. EAT KETO, CLEANER AND HEALTHIER
2. EXERCISE
3. LOVE MYSELF
4.
5.
6.
7.
8.
9.
10.

WORKOUT TRACKER

EXERCISE	REPS	SETS	WEIGHT	NOTES

HOW MANY HOURS OF SLEEP DID I GET? _____

BREAKFAST	LUNCH	DINNER

SNACKS

WATER

MACROS FOR THE DAY

CARBS: _____
PROTEIN: _____
FATS: _____
TOTAL CALORIES: _____

ENERGY LEVEL

MY GOALS

1. EAT KETO, CLEANER AND HEALTHIER
2. EXERCISE
3. LOVE MYSELF
4.
5.
6.
7.
8.
9.
10.

WORKOUT TRACKER

EXERCISE	REPS	SETS	WEIGHT	NOTES

HOW MANY HOURS OF SLEEP DID I GET? _____

BREAKFAST	**LUNCH**	**DINNER**

SNACKS

WATER

MACROS FOR THE DAY

CARBS: _____
PROTEIN: _____
FATS: _____
TOTAL CALORIES: _____

MY GOALS

1. EAT KETO, CLEANER AND HEALTHIER
2. EXERCISE
3. LOVE MYSELF
4.
5.
6.
7.
8.
9.
10.

ENERGY LEVEL

😀 😀 😐 😑 😴 💩

WORKOUT TRACKER

EXERCISE	REPS	SETS	WEIGHT	NOTES

DAY 72   **HOW MANY HOURS OF SLEEP DID I GET?** _____

| BREAKFAST | LUNCH | DINNER |

SNACKS

WATER

MACROS FOR THE DAY

CARBS: _____
PROTEIN: _____
FATS: _____
TOTAL CALORIES: _____

ENERGY LEVEL

😄 😊 😐 😒 😴 💩

MY GOALS

1. EAT KETO, CLEANER AND HEALTHIER
2. EXERCISE
3. LOVE MYSELF
4.
5.
6.
7.
8.
9.
10.

WORKOUT TRACKER

EXERCISE	REPS	SETS	WEIGHT	NOTES

BREAKFAST	LUNCH	DINNER

NACKS

ATER

ACROS FOR THE DAY

CARBS: _____
PROTEIN: _____
FATS: _____
TOTAL CALORIES: _____

NERGY LEVEL

MY GOALS

1. EAT KETO, CLEANER AND HEALTHIER
2. EXERCISE
3. LOVE MYSELF
4.
5.
6.
7.
8.
9.
10.

ORKOUT TRACKER

EXERCISE	REPS	SETS	WEIGHT	NOTES

HOW MANY HOURS OF SLEEP DID I GET? _____

BREAKFAST	LUNCH	DINNER

SNACKS

WATER

MACROS FOR THE DAY

CARBS: _____

PROTEIN: _____

FATS: _____

TOTAL CALORIES: _____

MY GOALS

1. EAT KETO, CLEANER AND HEALTHIER

2. EXERCISE

3. LOVE MYSELF

4.

5.

6.

7.

8.

9.

10.

ENERGY LEVEL

WORKOUT TRACKER

EXERCISE	REPS	SETS	WEIGHT	NOTES

HOW MANY HOURS OF SLEEP DID I GET? _____

BREAKFAST	LUNCH	DINNER

SNACKS

WATER

MACROS FOR THE DAY

CARBS: _____
PROTEIN: _____
FATS: _____
TOTAL CALORIES: _____

MY GOALS

1. EAT KETO, CLEANER AND HEALTHIER
2. EXERCISE
3. LOVE MYSELF
4.
5.
6.
7.
8.
9.
10.

ENERGY LEVEL

WORKOUT TRACKER

EXERCISE	REPS	SETS	WEIGHT	NOTES

DAY 76

BREAKFAST   LUNCH   DINNER

SNACKS

WATER

MACROS FOR THE DAY

CARBS: _____
PROTEIN: _____
FATS: _____
TOTAL CALORIES: _____

ENERGY LEVEL

MY GOALS

1. EAT KETO, CLEANER AND HEALTHIER
2. EXERCISE
3. LOVE MYSELF
4.
5.
6.
7.
8.
9.
10.

WORKOUT TRACKER

EXERCISE	REPS	SETS	WEIGHT	NOTES

BREAKFAST	**LUNCH**	**DINNER**

NACKS

VATER

MACROS FOR THE DAY

CARBS: _____

PROTEIN: _____

FATS: _____

TOTAL CALORIES: _____

MY GOALS

1. EAT KETO, CLEANER AND HEALTHIER

2. EXERCISE

3. LOVE MYSELF

4.

5.

6.

7.

8.

9.

10.

ENERGY LEVEL

WORKOUT TRACKER

EXERCISE	REPS	SETS	WEIGHT	NOTES

DAY 78

BREAKFAST	LUNCH	DINNER

SNACKS

WATER

MACROS FOR THE DAY
CARBS: _____
PROTEIN: _____
FATS: _____
TOTAL CALORIES: _____

ENERGY LEVEL

MY GOALS
1. EAT KETO, CLEANER AND HEALTHIER
2. EXERCISE
3. LOVE MYSELF
4.
5.
6.
7.
8.
9.
10.

WORKOUT TRACKER

EXERCISE	REPS	SETS	WEIGHT	NOTES

HOW MANY HOURS OF SLEEP DID I GET? _____

BREAKFAST	LUNCH	DINNER

SNACKS

WATER

MACROS FOR THE DAY

CARBS: _____
PROTEIN: _____
FATS: _____
TOTAL CALORIES: _____

MY GOALS

1. EAT KETO, CLEANER AND HEALTHIER
2. EXERCISE
3. LOVE MYSELF
4.
5.
6.
7.
8.
9.
10.

ENERGY LEVEL

WORKOUT TRACKER

EXERCISE	REPS	SETS	WEIGHT	NOTES

BREAKFAST	**LUNCH**	**DINNER**

SNACKS

WATER

MACROS FOR THE DAY

CARBS: _____

PROTEIN: _____

FATS: _____

TOTAL CALORIES: _____

ENERGY LEVEL

MY GOALS

1. EAT KETO, CLEANER AND HEALTHIER

2. EXERCISE

3. LOVE MYSELF

4.

5.

6.

7.

8.

9.

10.

WORKOUT TRACKER

EXERCISE	REPS	SETS	WEIGHT	NOTES

HOW MANY HOURS OF SLEEP DID I GET? _____

BREAKFAST	LUNCH	DINNER

NACKS

ATER

ACROS FOR THE DAY

CARBS: _____

PROTEIN: _____

FATS: _____

TOTAL CALORIES: _____

NERGY LEVEL

MY GOALS

1. EAT KETO, CLEANER AND HEALTHIER

2. EXERCISE

3. LOVE MYSELF

4.

5.

6.

7.

8.

9.

10.

ORKOUT TRACKER

EXERCISE	REPS	SETS	WEIGHT	NOTES

DAY 82   **HOW MANY HOURS OF SLEEP DID I GET?** _____

BREAKFAST	LUNCH	DINNER

SNACKS

WATER

MACROS FOR THE DAY

CARBS: _____

PROTEIN: _____

FATS: _____

TOTAL CALORIES: _____

ENERGY LEVEL

MY GOALS

1. EAT KETO, CLEANER AND HEALTHIER
2. EXERCISE
3. LOVE MYSELF
4.
5.
6.
7.
8.
9.
10.

WORKOUT TRACKER

EXERCISE	REPS	SETS	WEIGHT	NOTES

| BREAKFAST | LUNCH | DINNER |

SNACKS

WATER

MACROS FOR THE DAY

CARBS: _____
PROTEIN: _____
FATS: _____
TOTAL CALORIES: _____

ENERGY LEVEL

😄 😊 😐 😑 😴 💩

MY GOALS

1. EAT KETO, CLEANER AND HEALTHIER
2. EXERCISE
3. LOVE MYSELF
4.
5.
6.
7.
8.
9.
10.

WORKOUT TRACKER

EXERCISE	REPS	SETS	WEIGHT	NOTES

DAY 84

HOW MANY HOURS OF SLEEP DID I GET? _____

BREAKFAST

LUNCH

DINNER

SNACKS

WATER

MACROS FOR THE DAY

CARBS: _____
PROTEIN: _____
FATS: _____
TOTAL CALORIES: _____

ENERGY LEVEL

😊 😊 😕 😑 😴 💩

MY GOALS

1. EAT KETO, CLEANER AND HEALTHIER
2. EXERCISE
3. LOVE MYSELF
4.
5.
6.
7.
8.
9.
10.

WORKOUT TRACKER

EXERCISE	REPS	SETS	WEIGHT	NOTES

HOW MANY HOURS OF SLEEP DID I GET? _____

BREAKFAST	**LUNCH**	**DINNER**

SNACKS

WATER

MACROS FOR THE DAY

CARBS: _____

PROTEIN: _____

FATS: _____

TOTAL CALORIES: _____

ENERGY LEVEL

MY GOALS

1. EAT KETO, CLEANER AND HEALTHIER

2. EXERCISE

3. LOVE MYSELF

4.

5.

6.

7.

8.

9.

10.

WORKOUT TRACKER

EXERCISE	REPS	SETS	WEIGHT	NOTES

DAY 86

BREAKFAST	LUNCH	DINNER

SNACKS

WATER

MACROS FOR THE DAY

CARBS: _____
PROTEIN: _____
FATS: _____
TOTAL CALORIES: _____

ENERGY LEVEL

MY GOALS

1. EAT KETO, CLEANER AND HEALTHIER
2. EXERCISE
3. LOVE MYSELF
4.
5.
6.
7.
8.
9.
10.

WORKOUT TRACKER

EXERCISE	REPS	SETS	WEIGHT	NOTES

HOW MANY HOURS OF SLEEP DID I GET? _____

BREAKFAST	**LUNCH**	**DINNER**

SNACKS

WATER

MACROS FOR THE DAY

CARBS: _____

PROTEIN: _____

FATS: _____

TOTAL CALORIES: _____

ENERGY LEVEL

😃 😊 🙁 😑 😴 💩

MY GOALS

1. EAT KETO, CLEANER AND HEALTHIER
2. EXERCISE
3. LOVE MYSELF
4.
5.
6.
7.
8.
9.
10.

WORKOUT TRACKER

EXERCISE	REPS	SETS	WEIGHT	NOTES

DAY 88 HOW MANY HOURS OF SLEEP DID I GET? _____

BREAKFAST   LUNCH   DINNER

SNACKS

WATER

MACROS FOR THE DAY
CARBS: _____
PROTEIN: _____
FATS: _____
TOTAL CALORIES: _____

MY GOALS
1. EAT KETO, CLEANER AND HEALTHIER
2. EXERCISE
3. LOVE MYSELF
4.
5.
6.
7.
8.
9.
10.

ENERGY LEVEL

WORKOUT TRACKER

EXERCISE	REPS	SETS	WEIGHT	NOTES

BREAKFAST	LUNCH	DINNER

NACKS

ATER

ACROS FOR THE DAY

CARBS: _____

PROTEIN: _____

FATS: _____

TOTAL CALORIES: _____

NERGY LEVEL

MY GOALS

1. EAT KETO, CLEANER AND HEALTHIER

2. EXERCISE

3. LOVE MYSELF

4.

5.

6.

7.

8.

9.

10.

ORKOUT TRACKER

EXERCISE	REPS	SETS	WEIGHT	NOTES

HOW MANY HOURS OF SLEEP DID I GET? _____

BREAKFAST	LUNCH	DINNER

SNACKS

WATER

MACROS FOR THE DAY

CARBS: _____
PROTEIN: _____
FATS: _____
TOTAL CALORIES: _____

ENERGY LEVEL

MY GOALS

1. EAT KETO, CLEANER AND HEALTHIER
2. EXERCISE
3. LOVE MYSELF
4.
5.
6.
7.
8.
9.
10.

WORKOUT TRACKER

EXERCISE	REPS	SETS	WEIGHT	NOTES

LET'S NEVER GO BACK!
MEASUREMENTS

CHEST: _____

BICEP: _____

WAIST: _____

HIP: _____

THIGHS: _____

CALVES: _____

WEIGHT: _____

HEART RATE: _____

BLOOD PRESSURE: _____

LET'S NEVER GO BACK!
MEASUREMENTS

CHEST: _____

BICEP: _____

WAIST: _____

HIP: _____

THIGHS: _____

CALVES: _____

WEIGHT: _____

HEART RATE: _____

BLOOD PRESSURE: _____

NOTES

CPSIA information can be obtained
at www.ICGtesting.com
Printed in the USA
JSHW031454150720
6699JS00005B/28